This book is dedicated to all my friends and family who have supported me to become the man, the myth, the Future Doc House I am today. Special thanks first and foremost to my parents who loved me to a fault and raised me to become the man I am today. Thanks to my wife for tirelessly supporting and understanding the crazy late nights spent working on my projects. Thanks to my children for teaching me patience and unconditional love.

To my close friends: Damian Ratajczak, Barrington Kirkham, Agnieszka Szymczak, Michał Mazurek, Lasse Hodne, Dr. Ziya Aktig, Dr. Michaela Varys, and Dr. Kohei Yamada for always enthusiastically encouraging and supporting me.

Special mention to the Universities that have trained and educated me:

- Pepperdine University
- San Jose State University
- Notre Dame de Namur
- Charles University First Faculty of Medicine
- American University of Antigua
- Poznan University of Medical Science

Special mention to: Babcia, My in-laws, Nathan, Michał, Jonathan, Marco, Luis, Kamila, Hanna, Cristina, Jia, Mark, Howard, Kate, Zuza, Jessica, Angela, Alex, Gosia, RMS, Qupi Legacy Foundation, YouTube subscribers, and all my friends from Prague, Poland, California and around the world.

Finally, to those who I have failed to mention, you know who you are.

Is There a Doctor Aboard?

An Urgent Call for Change in Medical Education and Government Policy

By Future Doc House

ISBN 978-0-692-16523-2

Is There a Doctor Aboard?

An Urgent Call for Change in Medical Education and Government Policy

By Future Doc House

Table of Contents:

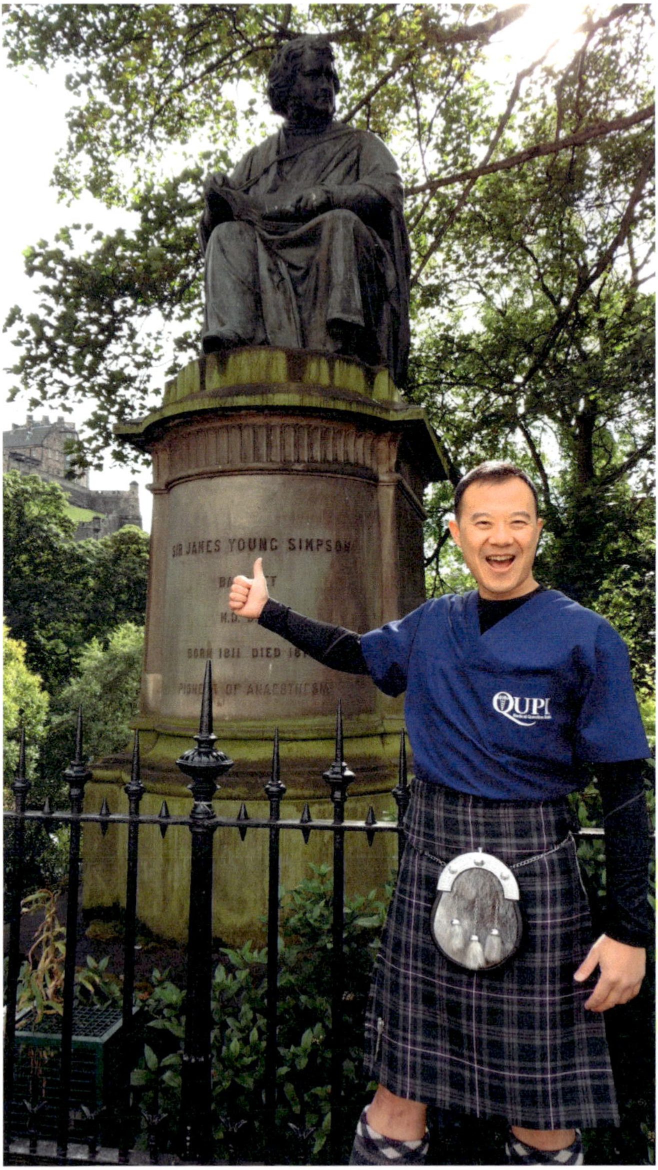

Future Doc House infront of the statue of
Dr. James Young Simpson in Scotland's Capital City, Edinburgh

Foreword

Dear Colleagues, Friends, and Supporters,

This book was written with no biased intentions and no political agenda. For I believe in life there are no true villains. We all do things for selfish reasons. We are born and instinctively we do what we need to survive. We need food so we grow it or get a job to pay for it. We need love so we keep our family close and seek out friends or lovers. We know our life is temporary so we create new life in the form of children—our progeny, our legacy. People think charitable foundations are a selfless act. I believe it is the most selfish act. The Qupi Legacy Foundation was created as a gift to the world for the selfish reason of wanting my life and legacy to serve a greater purpose than making and amassing a fortune I will not be able to spend when I die. So be selfish and know that we can do nothing for the past. The present is also now the past. So I only look toward the future.

Future Doc House

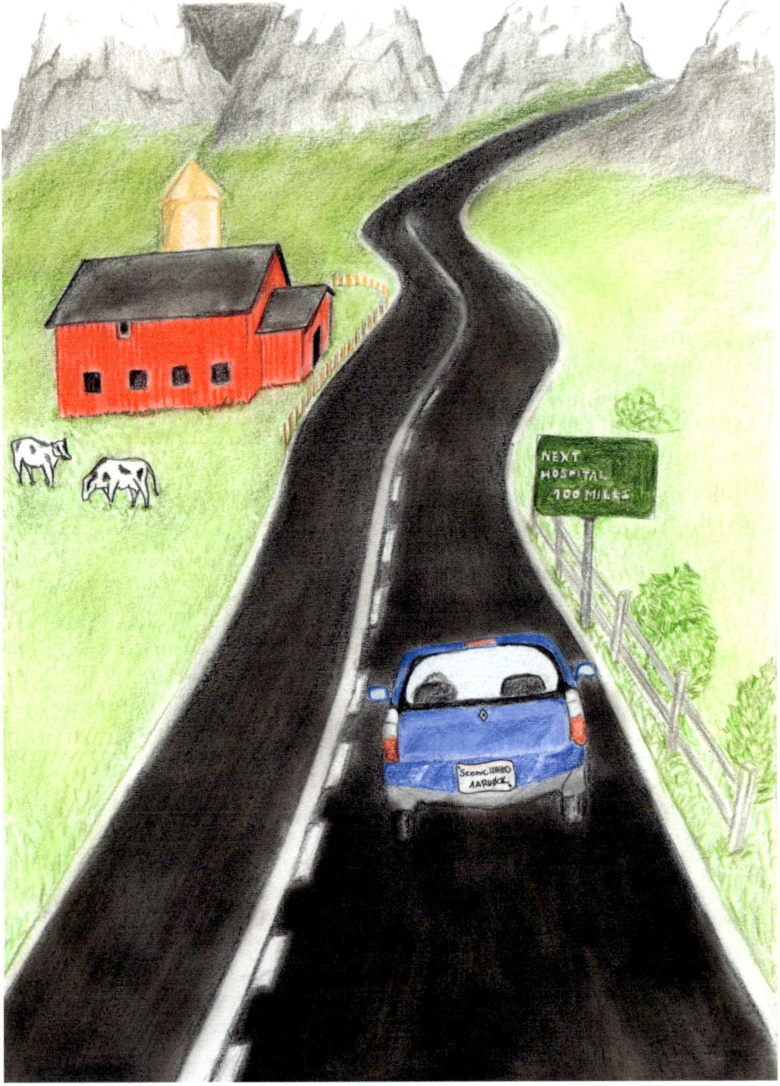
NEXT
HOSPITAL
100 MILES
Scenic IDAHO

Introduction: Do Not Get Sick in the United States of America

The United States of America remains the world's superpower. Despite being mired in controversy, it is still seen by much of the planet as a "shining city on the hill." Thirteen percent of the world's adults—or close to 700 million people—would move to the United States if they could, according to Gallup. But when they arrive, it might shock them to learn that medical care in the U.S. faces problems generally associated with the kinds of developing countries that most people want to emigrate from, not immigrate to.

The scene is a dire one: imagine a woman in a rural area, maybe in Tennessee, South Carolina or one of the other many states that the Human Services Health Resources Administration (HRSA) has designated as a "medically underserved area" because of its poor access to primary care. We'll call the woman in our example Jane.

Jane lives alone. She is elderly and retired with adult children living in distant cities, far away from her. She has enjoyed reasonably strong health and manages to get by on her own without too much struggle. However, the closest health clinic to her is a long drive away and has appalling wait times to see a doctor—so she hasn't seen a primary care physician in almost a year.

One morning Jane wakes up feeling short of breath, as if she has just climbed a flight of stairs. She experiences tightness in the chest, and begins to feel anxious. Of course, the anxiety only amplifies her breathing problems. The nearest hospital is fifty miles away, and she doesn't want to call an ambulance because she knows it would take a long time to arrive, and she isn't certain that her condition is serious. After all, she lives without any known health conditions.

Jane decides to wait. She masters her anxiety, and manages to get out of bed and brew a cup of tea in the kitchen. But throughout the morning, her symptoms worsen. She experiences severe trouble breathing. Finally, she decides to get in her car and drive the long, dusty highway toward town, and check herself in to the hospital.

By the time Jane arrives at the hospital, she parks her car and stumbles into the emergency room. Desperately short of breath, she knows her situation is serious. She's feeling light-headed and can't believe she made the long drive here without passing out.

Inside, Jane finds a scene of carnage such as one would expect to see in a developing country. Doctors and interns are running to and fro, wiping the sweat off their brows. People are being dragged in with horrific injuries from road accidents. One man appears to have wounded his leg with a chainsaw; another woman appears to be having an allergic reaction, her face puffy and swollen. Taking a number, Jane half collapses on a chair, and tries to close her

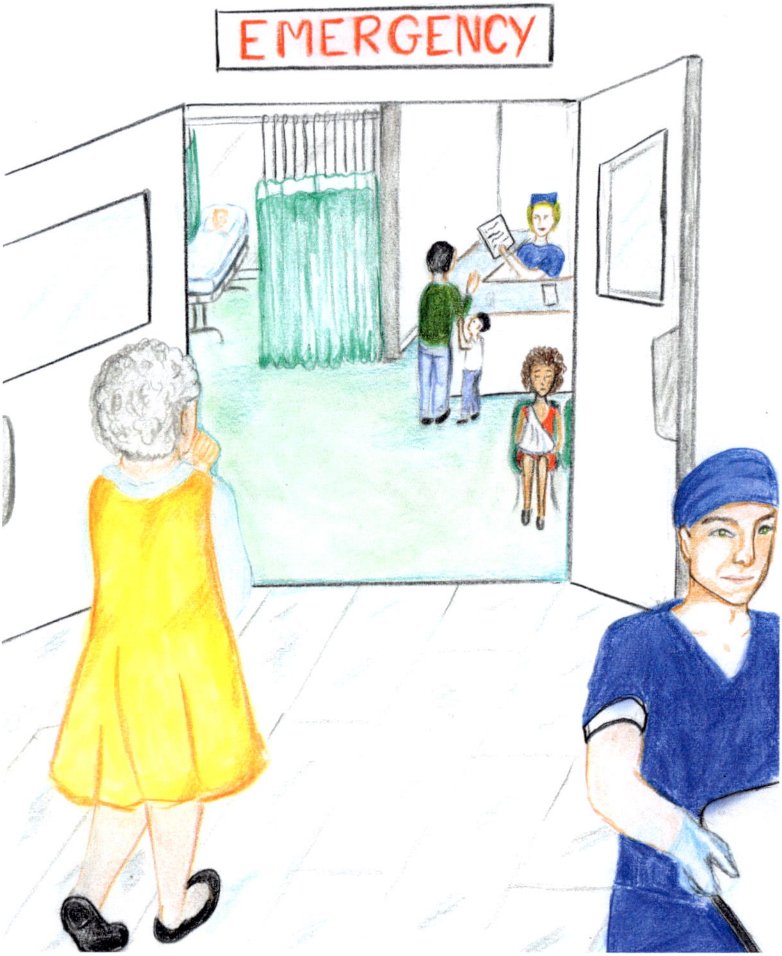
EMERGENCY

eyes and shut out the chaos surrounding her.

According to the Center for Disease Control, the U.S. sees 137 million emergency room visits per year. Hospitals are often understaffed and underfunded, so emergency room wait times can balloon to several hours or more. With harried staff and stretched resources, triage can be a delicate business, and those who require the most urgent care can be left waiting for dangerous lengths of time. We'll examine the root causes and break down the problem from an analytical perspective shortly. For now let's get back to Jane.

Jane's breath is coming in shorter and in more painful bursts, and the tightness in her chest continues to worsen and worsen. Finally, she is led in to see a doctor, who is accompanied by her young resident physician, Jeff.

It's only Jeff's second week on his ER rotation. He studied medicine in a big city in the next state over, but this was the only residency he was able to get. He left behind his friends, his family, and finds himself frequently working 12+ hour days in battle-ground conditions, struggling to keep up with the constant life-or-death challenges that seem to pile up with every second of each working day.

Jeff's supervisor is called away to attend to a family that was in a horrific car crash and has just been rushed into the emergency room, bleeding profusely. Jeff is left to deal with the situation alone. It's only mid afternoon, but already he's dead on his feet. He has a splitting headache and is dehydrated. The adrenaline that fueled him through the first few days of his job have been replaced by numbness and a sense of overwhelm. All he wants to do is sleep, but for the few hours he gets to spend in his bed at night he is kept awake by the horrific images that bombard him at work every day.

Jane is relieved to finally be receiving the attention of a doctor. Although Jeff looks young—and tired—she is sure that he wouldn't be in the hospital, wearing his uniform, if he weren't adequately trained and up for the job. But she is growing weak, and just wants her symptoms to be relieved so she can rest and recover.

The medical interview begins, and Jeff establishes a medical history and determines that Jane has no chronic conditions that she is aware of. While she is clearly suffering, she is conscious and breathing, and with the ER steadily filling up with patients who appear to be in far more obvious danger, he prescribes Jane some pills and sends her out the door.

Feeling a little miffed by the brusque treatment—after hours of waiting she was with a doctor for barely five minutes—and continuing to feel light-headed, Jane heads out. She'll visit the pharmacy, then drive back home and try to get some rest.

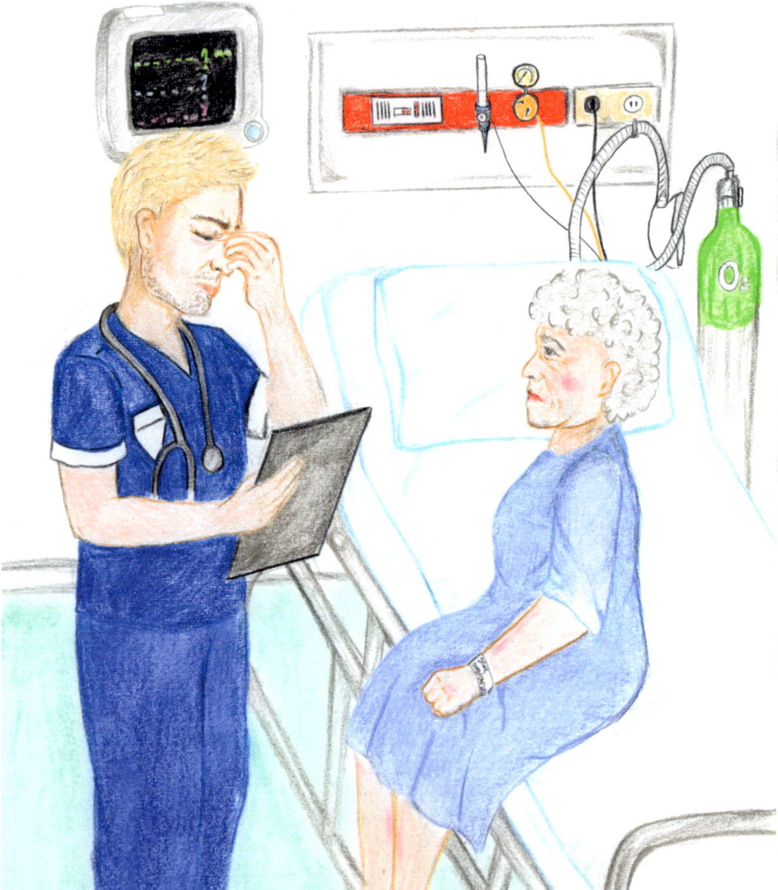
O_2

How shall we end this story?

Perhaps the shortness of breath causes Jane to collapse while driving on the highway, and she suffers a car crash, injuring or killing not just her, but other innocent lives as well. Perhaps she makes it home, but stops breathing in her sleep. Perhaps her symptoms were signs of a chronic condition which, left undiagnosed, will worsen over the coming months. Or perhaps she'll be fine. But are the odds really in her favor?

As we can see from this everyday and by no means "worst case" scenario, medical care in the U.S. is reaching crisis point:

- Hospitals are understaffed.
- Doctors are overworked.
- Patients are underserved.

The question now is not whether there is a problem. What needs to be asked is: How did we get here, and what can we do about it? These are the questions that this treatise sets out to answer.

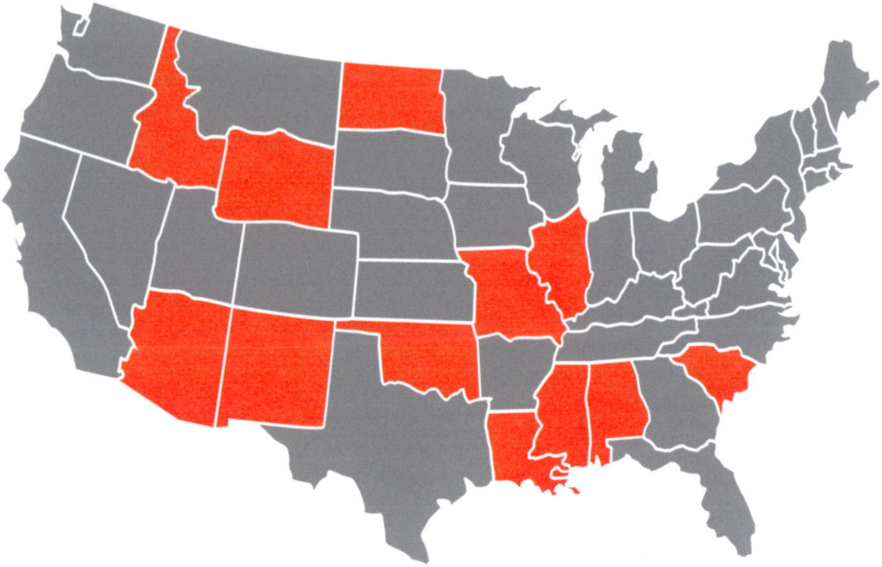

Medically undeserved areas
Source:
https://www.umhs-sk.org/blog/medically-underserved-areas-regions-where-u-s-needs-doctors/

The Root of the Problem: The U.S. Is Desperately Short of Doctors

Mark Twain wrote that only two things in life are inevitable: death and taxes. He may have added a third: a visit to the doctor. Young or old, rich or poor, we all require medical help throughout our lives. Without sufficient doctors, you simply cannot have a successful and thriving society. The health of the workforce, economic prosperity and people's ability to enjoy their lives absolutely depends on a strong healthcare system, adequately staffed by trained and qualified doctors.

It would be nice to rest in the belief that medical help will always be available when we need it. Particularly in the United States—the wealthiest and most powerful country the world has ever seen—it would be natural to assume that there are enough doctors to meet the needs of the population. Unfortunately, this is far from the case. The United States is heading toward a healthcare crisis, with an aging population placing unprecedented strain on an already overstretched medical system. Changes on the level of government and education are urgently required to address the problem.

The scale of the problem is almost as astonishing as the ease with which it could be solved. Outdated policies, a lumbering education system, and the ignorance of lawmakers have put America in a dangerous situation which they can and must get out of.

Here's how things stand today: TechCrunch, citing a recent study by the American Association of Medical Colleges, reports that by 2025, the U.S. could lack as many as 35,600 primary care physicians. While this guide will focus mostly on the U.S., this problem is not limited to North America. Globally speaking, we're already short 7.2 million healthcare workers with that number expected to rise to almost 13 million within the next two decades, according to the World Health Organization.

Millions of Americans already live in areas without sufficient healthcare. These so-called 'medically underserved areas' include the entire states of Alabama, Arizona, Idaho, Illinois, Louisiana, Mississippi, Missouri, New Mexico, North Dakota, Oklahoma, South Carolina and Wyoming!

When you travel through America, you notice that every town has a police station. Every town has a fire station. Every town has a church. But many towns lack their own hospitals. Doctors prefer to work in urban areas. This adds up to long and often expensive journeys to receive medical care for the ill, who too often fail to get the attention they so badly require.

While most Americans suffer, Native Americans in particular feel invisible in the current healthcare system. With life expectancy for Native Americans up to 20 years lower than the national average in many states, it is clear that their communities are in serious need of improved health care services. In conversation with NPR, Native American nurse Margaret Moss explained just how insufficient this current service is. Describing a physician incorrectly setting the arm of a Native American patient, Moss is reported as saying, "Even when I, as an [medically] educated person using the right words, was saying what needed to happen, [he] didn't want to do anything for us, even though we had a [health insurance] card."

While most of the issues discussed in this document are political, financial and systemic, the example of Margaret Moss points to a level of callousness that hides below the surface of much of America's healthcare system. Here is a doctor being told by an expert that he was incorrectly setting the arm of a patient—potentially crippling that patient for life and certainly causing lasting and unnecessary pain—and the doctor appeared to lack the compassion or empathy to correct his mistake.

One can easily understand Moss's fury at this injustice, and empathize with the hurt and frustration—not to mention actual physical pain—of the Native American patient involved. It is tempting to write off the doctor in Moss's example as a one-off bad egg. It could—perhaps justifiably—be blamed on racism. But such issues are not one-offs, and condemning an individual doctor we don't know offhand does not help us solve the wider problems.

As we will explore in detail later, the process of training doctors in the U.S. frequently results in depressed, emotionally damaged MDs who are well trained in medical knowledge, but lack the human skills of empathy and compassion which patients so desperately need.

This is not something that can be changed quickly. Training a doctor takes a long time, so as the Association of American Medical Colleges (AAMC) puts it, a 2015 problem is actually a 2025 problem. Things are already bad, and set to get progressively worse year over year. As of 2018, we're still far from putting in place the systemic changes required to address this problem. But this is something that can be changed. A solution is not outside the capacity of the U.S. government, nor is it beyond the reach of the largest economy on Earth.

While these statistics can seem abstract, the consequences of the doctor shortage are immediate, and already being felt across the U.S. In 2017, Forbes reported that doctor wait times had soared 30%. Across the country it takes an average of 24 days to get an appointment with a physician, but worse is yet to come. In places like Boston, where the average doctor wait time is already at a staggering 52 days, we're getting a preview of where things may be heading if rapid changes aren't made.

Most of the news is bad, but there are promising signs. New technology is improving the accessibility of medicine and the speed and efficiency of medical education. The doctor shortage is becoming mainstream news, with coverage from CBS and the Washington Post within the last few years. The doctor shortage is now a well established fact, but will the government and the nation's educational institutions take sufficient action in time?

Before we can prescribe a solution, we first need to diagnose the causes of the problem. Unfortunately, the primary cause is a factor beyond anyone's control: an aging population. It is perhaps ironic that because of 20th century improvements in medicine, people are living longer, meaning the very same medical system that achieved such staggering advances is now unable to cope with the increased strain. The number of Americans 65 and over is already a staggering 46 million! This number is expected to exceed 98 million by 2060. It should be overwhelmingly clear already that we're heading at high speed toward a national health catastrophe.

Other factors contributing to the doctor shortage could easily be solved by more intelligent policy making. For example, one in four doctors currently practicing in America is foreign born. Many of whom are citizens, others are immigrants who travel to the U.S. to provided valuable skills. Unfortunately, instead of embracing the help from overseas that the U.S. desperately needs, politicians like Donald Trump exacerbate the problem with travel bans and visa restrictions, keeping up to 1,000 qualified and hardworking doctors per year out of the country. Meanwhile, citizens desperately wait for medical attention. Immigration restrictions could be reversed by a change of government, but there's nothing we can do to stop our population from aging. There are, however, actions we can take to mitigate the cost to our society. This broadly comes down to three areas:

- Government policy
- Corporate action
- Education

All three areas require rethinking to face the realities of the current situation in the U.S. This manifesto will present a broad plan for all three areas, focused toward one goal: solving the doctor shortage first in the United States, and then in the world at large. We cannot stop the population from aging, but we can lift restrictions and streamline the education process, creating more doctors who are trained and equipped to combat the problem.

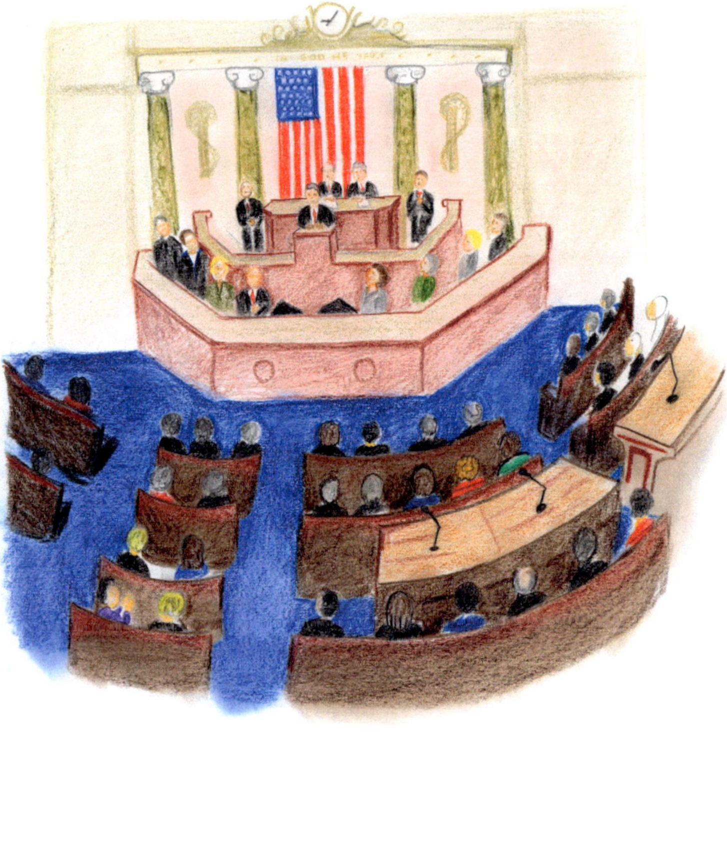

How Government Policy Could Provide the Change Needed

The fact that the U.S. is facing a major doctor shortage is to a large extent the fault of government policy. Caps on federally funded residency programs mean that too few Americans have the opportunity to train and qualify as doctors. Training a doctor is a long and arduous process. As older doctors retire and an aging population puts ever increasing strain on the medical system, the ratio of doctors to patients creeps ever lower.
The AAMC lives with this problem every day, and has announced its specific policy recommendations to begin alleviating the doctor shortage. Examining the material on their website, we can see that the AAMC broadly has two policy priorities with regard to the doctor shortage:

1. To reduce federal caps on residency that are preventing new doctors from entering the workforce.

2. To better support and fund public service programs like the National Health Service Corps (NHSC) and Public Service Loan Forgiveness (PSLF) that make it easier for institutions to recruit and retain physicians.

Let's look at both these aims in more detail, using details from the AAMC policy documents as cited above.

Lifting Federal Residency Caps

While medical school enrollments are up an impressive 30% across the U.S. at large, Medicare support for graduate residency programs has remained locked in place since 1997! This means that while many students have the intelligence and ambition to become doctors, the financial support to make it possible for them to complete their training and enter the workforce simply isn't there. This is an imbalance that urgently needs to be addressed.

As the St. Louis Post-Dispatch succinctly puts it:

"Currently, the only way to become a practicing doctor in the U.S. is to complete a residency program after medical school. The problem is that for the past two decades there has been a cap on the number of residents funded by Medicare, which is the primary source of payment for residents."

These Medicare resident caps "limit the ability of teaching hospitals and medical schools to respond to the physician needs of their communities and the nation." A bill before Congress (H.R.2267) is already under consideration. It would go a long way toward fixing this problem by gradually increasing the number of residency slots nationally by 3,000 each year between 2019 and 2023, with a total increase of 15,000 slots.

This bill was introduced on introduced May 1, 2017 by Representatives Joseph

 Crowley (D-NY) and Ryan Costello (R-PA). You can read more about it and the reasons for the AAMC's support at:

https://aamc-black.global.ssl.fastly.net/production/media/filer_public/8a/00/8a00c0c5-354e-4545-a993-ee94a0acd64a/hr_2267_the_resident_physician_shortage_reduction_act_of_2017.pdf

The funding trail ultimately ends with teaching hospitals, the importance of which we'll discuss in the education chapter to come.

While state governments and private insurance companies pay for some residencies, the majority of funding comes from Medicare and Medicaid. According to the nonprofit Student Doctor Net, "This money eventually makes its way to the over 1,000 teaching hospitals where medical students go to serve as residents and hone their clinical skills. The cost however, is high: $9.5 billion from Medicare and an additional $2 billion in Medicaid annually. This money funds the 115,000 medical residents operating in the U.S. each year. The total cost breaks down to around $100,000 per year per resident."

This is a high financial burden for the government, but one that is absolutely integral for maintaining a functional healthcare system.

Making It Real: Life as a Medical Resident

All of us who've watched medical dramas on TV know about the grueling life of a medical resident. With funding caps in place, the number of medical graduates is set to outpace the number of residency slots available.

The state of medical care in the U.S. is already dire. As Student Doctor Net breaks it down:

- "60 million Americans lack access to regular primary care."
- "In the last 50 years, the percentage of primary care physicians has decreased from 50% to 30% of all practicing doctors."
- "1 in 5 patients who visit the ER could have had their problem resolved by a primary care physician."

Given these facts, surely we need to be supporting, encouraging and funding those medical students who are brave enough to give it their all at the residency stage. After all, life as a medical resident at one of the 1000+ teaching hospitals in the U.S. is no picnic.

Dr. Patrick Wiita, an intern at Los Angeles County/USC Medical Center, described a typical day of his to U.S. News & World Report.

In his hour-by-hour breakdown, he describes his second alarm going off at 5 AM. He sees his first patients at 6:30—grumpy kids who don't want to be there. Work, including seeing patients, doing rounds, and completing seemingly endless amounts of paperwork, continues for the next 12 hours!

Not until 7:30 PM—almost 15 hours after that second alarm went off—does the exhausted intern get to begin the journey home.

Many students are only accepted into residencies far from home. They leave behind their support network of friends and family, and the familiar comforts that they spent their whole lives growing up around. Because of their grueling schedules, they have little time to socialize. Old friends are far away and there simply isn't time to make new ones.
Rates of depression and suicide among junior doctors are sky high. And yet, each year, as many as 50,000 students apply to medical school in the U.S. alone. These people want to grow up to help others, to save lives, maybe even to help contribute to a cure for cancer.

Surely the government should have their backs, wouldn't you think?

To Increase Funding of Essential Public Services

In addition to the urgent need for the U.S. government to increase Medicare caps and fund more medical students to participate in federally funded residency programs, there are other actions that the government can take now to help more students graduate as doctors and enter the workforce, stethoscope in hand.

Becoming a doctor is an exceedingly expensive endeavor, with medical students amassing staggering amounts of debt. It is the norm—not the exception—for students across the U.S. to leave school with well over $200,000 of debt tied to their necks. The AAMC and the National Association of Student Financial Aid Administrators both recommend that caps on student loan forgiveness be increased so that they are at least level with the aggregate graduate and professional student loan limit (which sits at $224,000 for physicians).

This would relieve some of the horrifying financial pressure on medical students, allowing more students from less wealthy backgrounds to enter the medical profession and give back to their communities. Another essential program helping to relieve the financial burden on medical students is the National Health Service Corps. The NHSC provides loan repayment to physicians practicing medicine in communities with limited access to medical care—the very communities discussed earlier, which are already affected by the national doctor shortage.

The NHSC currently receives $310 million in mandatory federal funding every year, though this amount is not always guaranteed and the NHSC faces frequent moments of financial peril. The AAMC recommends a significant improvement of funding for the NHSC by both increasing the mandatory federal amount, as well as allowing additional funding for the Service Corps via annual appropriations. This will result in more financial support and incentives for doctors to work in rural areas, bringing medical care and attention to the communities who need it most desperately.

As things currently stand, 60 million primary care patients are currently unserved by physicians across the country at large. By lifting Medicare federal residency caps, lifting caps on loan forgiveness, and increasing funding for the NHSC, the U.S. government can take immediate and profound steps to address the need of these neglected patients.

The Insurance Crisis and How One Man Is Attempting to Solve It

The doctor shortage is, of course, not the whole story when it comes to the American healthcare crisis. It underpins the focus of this guide, and we will see how it is intricately connected to every aspect of healthcare from education to costs. However, it would be neglectful to pretend that the doctor shortage and the associated legislative shortcomings outlined above were the root of all problems facing the American people.

More than 28 million Americans currently lack insurance coverage, while millions more citizens live in medically underserved areas, facing huge costs and long wait times for even the most routine treatment. The issue of insurance coverage is divisive, and deeply entrenched in the political divide. The only thing Americans can seem to agree on is the simple fact that there is a problem, and that dramatic change is required if the citizens of the world's most powerful nation are to receive the medical care that they need.

As Americans become increasingly disillusioned with the sluggish pace of political change, powerful figures from outside the current administration have been working on their own solutions. As an example, we will focus briefly on Andy Slavitt.

From March 2015 to January 2017, Andy Slavitt was Acting Administrator of the Centers for Medicare and Medicaid Services (CMS), a position to which he was nominated by former President Barack Obama. After leaving office, Slavitt spent a year traveling the United States and talking to ordinary Americans about how the current healthcare deadlock is affecting their lives.

In an Op-Ed in *USA Today*, Slavitt wrote:

"Talk to a mom of a chronically ill child or a young man working in a fast food job without benefits, or a dad who lost his job and his insurance. Talking to Americans about their health care is often a conversation marked by vulnerability, fear, and the fragility of middle-class life."

To provide new ideas, policy support, and creative energy aimed at tackling America's healthcare crisis, Slavitt has unveiled his own nonpartisan initiative: United States of Care.

Announcing the initiative on Twitter on February 6, 2018, Slavitt wrote: "Today launches a new movement to attempt to get past the politics and get affordable care for every American. The work is just beginning and we need everyone to participate to change things."

The United States of Care's website, UnitedStatesofCare.org, outlines the organization's three guiding principles, which are:

- Affordable Source of Care: Every American should have an affordable regular source of care for themselves and their families.

- Protection from Financial Devastation: All Americans should be protected from financial devastation because of illness or injury.

- Political and Economic Viability: Policies to achieve these aims must be fiscally responsible and win the political support needed to ensure long-term stability.

As reported by *MedCity News*, Slavitt has already assembled an impressive group of well-known individuals to support his initiative, including Atul Gawande and former Kentucky Governor Steve Beshear, Dignity Health CEO Lloyd Dean, former Congresswoman Gabrielle Giffords, former CMS Deputy Administrator Patrick Conway, Allina Health CEO Penny Wheeler and Providence St. Joseph Health CEO Rod Hochman, as well as actors Bradley Whitford and Andy Richter, and astronaut Mark Kelly.

United States of Care has received mixed responses from the media. While the group strives to be above politics, the state of healthcare is already so mired in political entanglements that overcoming the political stalemate may be too much of a challenge, especially for a group started by someone who is often seen as an establishment figure closely associated with Obamacare, rather than an unaffiliated outsider.

The official blog of Physicians for a National Health Program, writes: "This organization that professes to place itself above politics is already smothered in anti-single-payer politics and is doomed to fail. Sad."

As a liberal activist, Slavitt has come under fire for supposedly abandoning politics in favor of a bipartisan approach. Some democrats fear that this is giving up, and maybe even handing a political victory to the republicans. Rather than carrying on the fight for liberal and democratic principles, some view Slavitt's initiative as an attempt to leave the battleground and pursue solutions elsewhere.

In an interview with CNN, Slavitt responds to this line of criticism: "The reality is that right now we don't have the political makeup where people have the incentive to compromise. We have people in a world where their incentive is to get more polarized. So when we say healthcare over politics is a top priority, it (means) that we want to have an impact on constituents first in making care accessible to all Americans."

Slavitt has been active on Twitter since launching the United States of Care, and while his organization may be nonpartisan, he himself doesn't seem to hide or obfuscate his political leanings.

In a Tweet posted April 7 with regard to the current midterm elections, he wrote, "Anything but a Democratic majority gives Trump free reign to take people's health care." Clearly, politics are not so easy to escape!

It is clear that, despite his experience and connections, Andy Slavitt has an enormous challenge in front of him if he wants to cut through the political stalemate and actually impel real change. While we agree strongly with the aims of his initiative, it remains to be seen whether or not this particular venture will live up to its aspirations.

While we welcome all positive initiatives, and government action is absolutely necessary, the government alone cannot solve the problem. We look now toward the corporate and educational sectors to examine what else is being done, and what can be done, across the broader spectrum of American society.

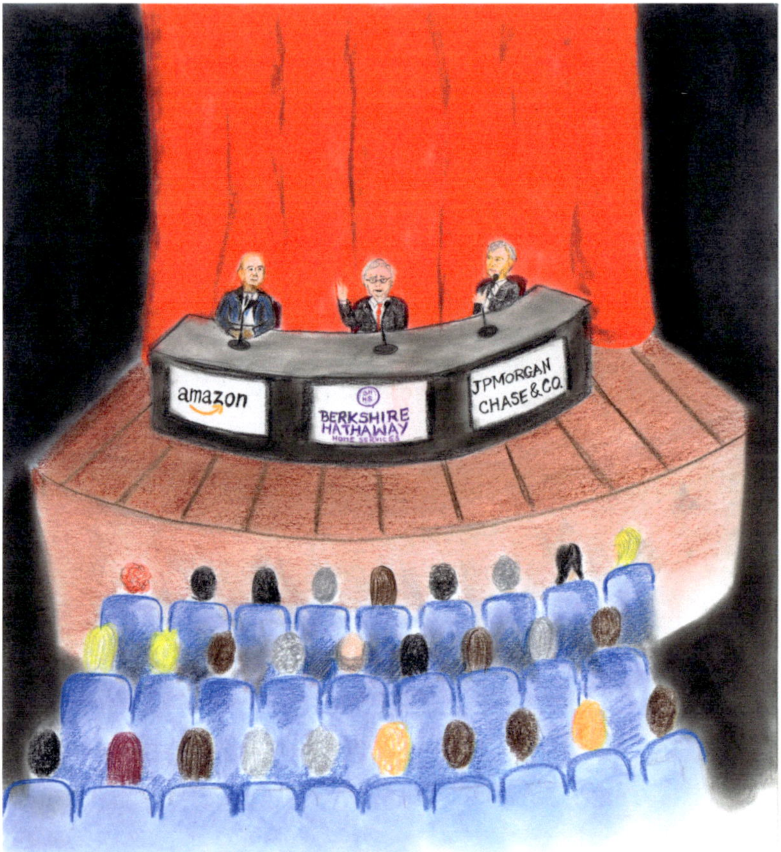
amazon
BERKSHIRE
HATHAWAY
HOME SERVICES
JPMORGAN
CHASE & CO.

How Corporate Giants Are Attempting to Change Healthcare in America

Medical costs and associated insurance premiums are skyrocketing. As reported by CNN, the Health Care Cost Institute reveals that total spending per person has risen 15% between 2012 and 2016 alone. Over the same time period, prescription drugs rose in cost by 25%.

Many of these costs are met by the corporations who pay a large portion of the healthcare insurance costs of their employees. Unsurprisingly, the power players are battling back. In January 2018, CNN Money reported that Jeff Bezos, Warren Buffett and Jamie Dimon—the leaders of Amazon, Berkshire Hathaway and JPMorgan Chase respectively—are teaming up to combat the skyrocketing healthcare costs for their combined 840,000 employees.

These companies have recently announced Atul Gawande as the CEO of their joint venture, and aim to slash healthcare costs by 15-20%. It is clear that their ambitions go beyond their own backyard. With their financial clout and—particularly in the case of Amazon—reputation for innovation, it's certainly possible that we'll be seeing some positive changes in the not-too-distant future.

However, there are reasons to temper our optimism. First and foremost, corporations are by nature self-interested. While they may act in the benefit of their communities, altruism only goes so far. It is hard to imagine that members of the poorer rural communities as discussed above are high on the priorities list for the likes of JPMorgan Chase. Another potential twist is that when healthcare is controlled by one's employer, the company has a vested interest to keep costs low. One could speculate that this may have negative results, such as employers screening new hires for their healthcare history.

A second reason to temper our optimism is that even the most innovative corporate solution to rising healthcare costs would only examine the surface of the issue. Unless Buffett, Bezos and Dimon are planning to lobby Congress to increase federal residency caps and provide financial relief for trainee doctors in underserved communities, the root causes of America's doctor shortage crisis will remain in place.

A Solution from Within the Medical Industry?

Amazon, Berkshire Hathaway and JPMorgan Chase look at healthcare from outside the industry. But what about those companies that exist in that world, employ doctors, create medical products, and are directly responsible for millions of patients, not just their own employees?

 An interesting case study is the venerable HMO giant, Kaiser Permanente. Kaiser has invested more than $10 billion over the last 15 years in technology to better coordinate patient care, meaning that better use can be made of the doctors and resources available. They themselves employ 17,000 salaried doctors across their 37 hospitals, giving them the power to streamline their own expenses as well as consolidate the care they deliver to clients. As reported by the New York Times, this integrated model is gaining favor with other hospitals across the country forming accountable care organizations (ACOs) by buying physician practices or partnering with doctors and health insurers.

This integrated approach is showing promise, but some experts—like Dr. Robert Berenson of the Urban Institute—caution against concentrating too much power in the hands of one institution. Kaiser's reach is also by no means perfect, with many patients in less served regions having to travel to different locations for surgery and to receive medication, causing stress as well as additional, unwelcome expense. n agency in California has also criticized Kaiser for having long wait times for mental health services. Kaiser says they are working on this.

Looking at the situation as it stands, we can see the Kaiser model as flawed but promising. By concentrating resources and taking responsibility to provide the technology, medicine, venue and—most importantly—physicians to its patients, integrated providers are capable of providing highly efficient services. However, if the legislative and educational barriers toward training enough new doctors persist, even the most efficient corporate or HMO structure will not be sufficient to provide adequate healthcare to all Americans.

While we celebrate any attempt to improve the condition for the average citizen, it is unwise to sit on our haunches and expect a corporate miracle to solve this problem. Americans are right to trust innovation—but this crisis can only be addressed with corporations, the government and the nation's educational institutions acting in lock-step. Let us now turn to education.

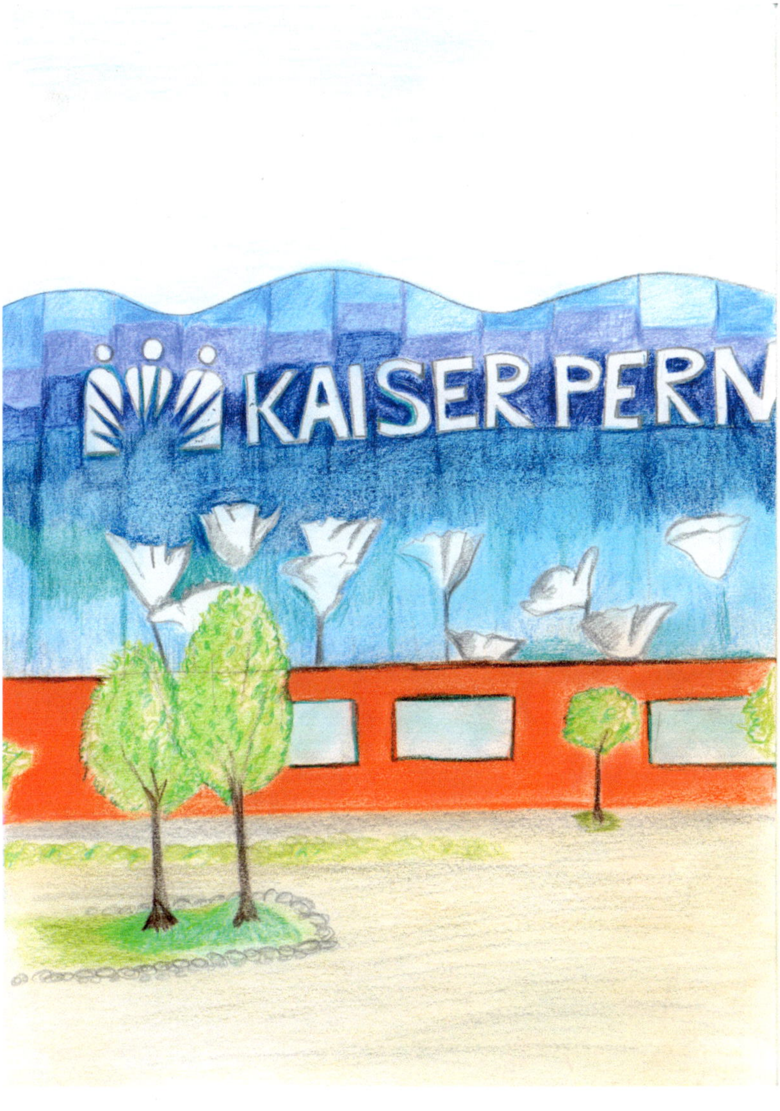
KAISER PERM

The Essential Role of Teaching Hospitals in the United States of America

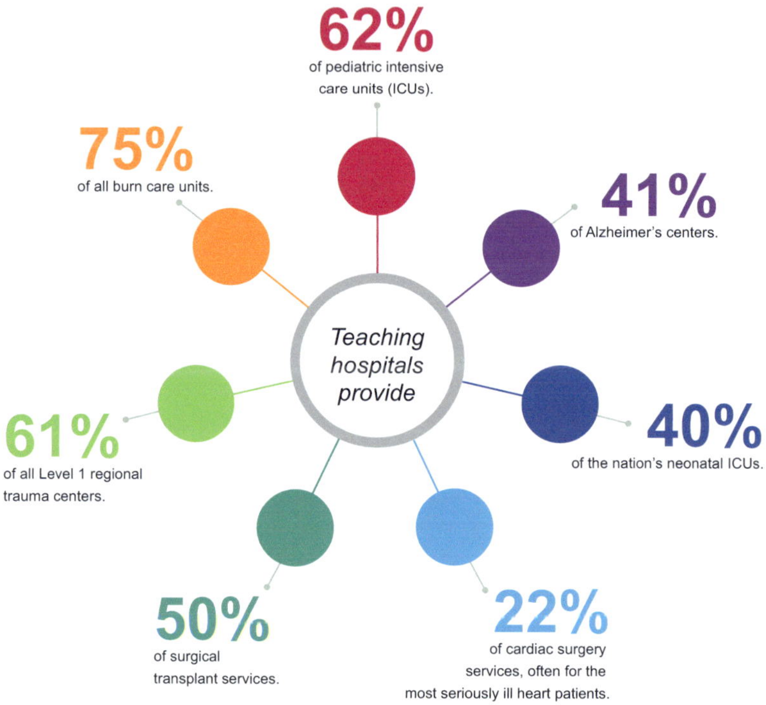

Source: AAMC.org

Education—Academia of Medicine Needs to Adapt

We saw above how federal funding caps on residency programming are preventing medical students from completing their studies and becoming doctors. We've looked at the problem from the perspective of government. Now we'll zoom in closer and look at this specifically on the level of Graduate Medical Education. As the AAMC puts it:

"With our nation facing a serious shortage of between 61,700 and 94,700 physicians by 2025, any number of medical students who do not have the opportunity to complete residency training is a serious concern. Academic medicine is rising to the challenge."

In 2016, as reported by CNN, 18,000 graduating MDs in the U.S. applied for close to 28,000 first-year residency positions. This means that the remaining 10,000 residencies were filled by foreign students lucky enough to obtain a visa. It is clear that academic medicine is not at present sufficiently funded or equipped to support American medical students through the whole course of their studies.

In addition to contributing to the nation's doctor shortage, the lack of American medical students reaching the residency stage has other consequences. Medicare pays the salaries of most residents at teaching hospitals across the U.S. Teaching hospitals have been described as the "economic engine" of many small towns, an essential piece of infrastructure that keeps the city both healthy and educated. Were these institutions to close, it would result in drastic consequences for the community.

As the AAMC outlines in detail, teaching hospitals don't just provide tomorrow's doctors. They provide essential care today. Despite making up just 6% of America's hospitals, teaching hospitals have a high level of sophistication that means they provide a disproportionate amount of essential care to the community, including:

- 75 percent of all burn care units;
- 62 percent of pediatric intensive care units (ICUs);
- 61 percent of all Level 1 regional trauma centers;
- 50 percent of surgical transplant services;
- 41 percent of Alzheimer's centers;
- 40 percent of the nation's neonatal ICUs; and
- 22 percent of cardiac surgery services, often for the most seriously ill heart patients.

At their best, teaching hospitals are where the highest virtues of academia and medicine combine. While some decry the high cost to the taxpayer and patient, David Silbersweig, Chairman of the Department of Psychiatry and Co-Director of the Institute for the Neurosciences at Brigham and Women's Hospital, and

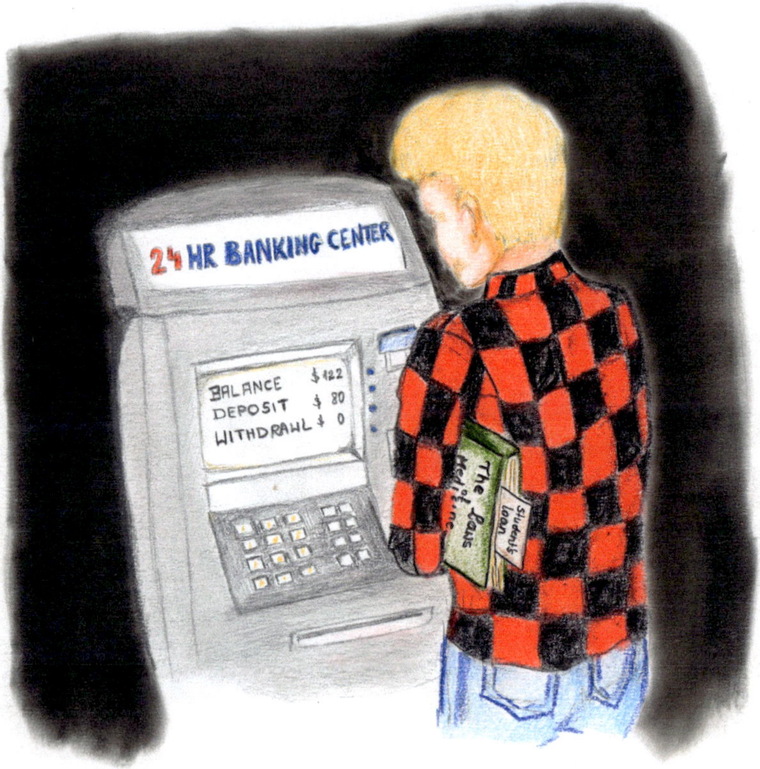

24 HR BANKING CENTER
BALANCE $122
DEPOSIT $ 80
WITHDRAWL $ 0
The Laws of
Students loan

Stanley Cobb, Professor of Psychiatry and Academic Dean (Partners HealthCare) at Harvard Medical School, provided an eloquent, even heartfelt, defense of the institution in a recent Washington Post article:

> "A different paradigm is needed. One in which there is an acknowledgment that it is the academics that underlie the clinical excellence of the teaching hospital. One in which there is not a disconnect or a zero-sum scenario between the clinical mission (with its economic imperatives) and the academic mission. One that views academic medical centers as health and wealth generators in the community, worthy of investment if not support."

It is clear that teaching hospitals will not endure at their current strength if they lack funding for the graduate students who provide such an integral part of their makeup. In addition to the government solutions proposed above that would increase funding for students and residency programs, there are other creative solutions that would better enable American medical students to reach the residency phase, contribute their time and expertise to teaching hospitals, and eventually graduate as fully qualified physicians.

We look now to technology:

Education Is Expensive—Are There More Efficient Ways This Can Be Done?

Too few American students are reaching the residency stage because of the high cost and lack of government funding. We saw above how medical students in the U.S. leave school with an average of $200,000+ in debt. It costs between $207,866 and $278,455 to send a student through medical school. As the efficiency of education and educational technology have increased, these costs have merely gone up, rather than going down.

Making It Real: The High Cost of Medical Education

CBS MoneyWatch asks whether medical school could be a $1 million mistake. Yes, doctors are paid well and account for the majority of 6-figure salaried jobs in the U.S. Orthopedic surgeons typically pull in more than $400,000 per year. But there are costs, too.

Many doctors across the U.S. have seen their pay decline in recent years. Bureaucratic interference has meant that the paperwork element—always a fact of any doctor's life—has dramatically escalated in recent years, and now accounts for one quarter of the average physician's time. It also takes up to 14 years to train a doctor. That is time that, in other professions, could be spent earning money and climbing the ladder.

Of course, most medical students don't enter the profession in order to simply get rich. Being a doctor is a noble calling, and can give ordinary people the chance to literally save lives. Given the importance of doctors and the fact that the U.S. desperately needs more of them, it is worth taking a further look at the high cost of medical education and how this affects real people.

On the website KevinMD, Dr. Cory S. Fawcett explains how, despite being financially cautious and working throughout much of his time as a medical student, he still ended up with close to half a million dollars in student debt. This debt went on to have major consequences throughout the rest of his life, as he explains:

"I had a bad case of 'debtabetic' neuropathy. I had spent so much time during my training with debt that I did not need to deal with, that I became numb to the consequences of debt. It was so easy to just borrow more money when I needed it. No payments until years later and no interest was accumulating. It doesn't get much easier than that. I fell headlong into the American way of using debt to finance my lifestyle."

While debt can seem like an abstract concept, its psychological consequences are real. People enter med school to become doctors and help others. Often they are left emotionally and financially broken, and are unable even to help themselves.

Of course, this is not an issue that affects only medical students. The website StudentDebtCrisis.org collects stories of how student debt has damaged lives across the U.S. What makes medical school particularly pernicious is the high length of study—with it taking between 10 and 14 years to become a doctor, there's more opportunity to acquire much larger amounts of debt before entering the workforce.

But there is hope. Services like the Public Service Loan Forgiveness (PSLF) Program can help free students from this burden. As one student, Megan, explains:

"I have been struggling to pay my student loans for years. But with the PSLF program,at least I know there is light at the end of the tunnel. Without an Income Driven Repayment Plan, I would be homeless. This program is ESSENTIAL to get qualified people to work in government and nonprofit sectors."

This is a problem that can be solved. The key is increased government support,including a greater flexibility and willingness to experiment with new teaching styles and to streamline the education system.

Thanks to the internet, information has never been more abundant. A student sitting at home in Washington State can stream a lecture from a professor at Yale or Princeton. Online education platforms employ principles like gamification to make learning more enjoyable and increase retention and comprehension. Online discussion forums allow students to discuss symptoms both obscure and common, and share their findings with their peers across the world.

Technology has already greatly increased the efficiency of medical practice. Telemedicine allows patients to connect with a doctor remotely. It's now commonplace for patients with a medical problem to use an app like Pager to efficiently summon a qualified doctor to their home—saving them a risky and expensive trip to an overcrowded hospital. If we now have an Uber for doctors, why does medical education today remain rooted firmly in the classrooms and confined to the dog-eared pages of clunky textbooks? Surely there is a more efficient way.

The opportunities afforded by technology have been toyed with by medical universities that use the internet to supplement their programs. Online education is now mainstream in many fields, and is an efficient, low-cost and recognized way for people to attain many forms of professional qualifications, from nursing to speech-language therapy. But no medical school in America has taken the plunge to go completely online.

There are a few natural reasons for this—for example, the high-stakes aspect of the profession that justifies its regulation, or by necessity, the hands-on-nature of many aspects of medical learning. But as any medical school will tell you, 90% of their time is spent with the textbooks or in the library, memorizing convoluted facts, processes and systems. This entire element of education could easily be moved online for many students with no loss of learning quality. For elements in which face-to-face interaction is necessary, periodic meetings or excursions could be arranged. The result of this would be a much cheaper way to educate students as doctors, without reducing the knowledge or skill level of online graduates.

By providing the option of online medical education, we can get more American students up to the residency stage with less cost. This means more doctors in teaching hospitals in the medium term, and more doctors in America in the long term.

Making It Real: American's First Online Medical University?

The idea of an online medical university is ridiculous to many. But is it really that insane?

The internet is already used to supplement medical education. With lectures from universities being streamed online and apps that help students study, it is an accepted argument that the internet can enhance and contribute to the learning process. Many schools are embracing information technology as an important tool to help students learn. Vanderbilt School of Medicine even redesigned their entire IT infrastructure to be inline with their new curriculum.

It seems the argument is won that technology like the internet can help medical students. But it still takes 10-14 years to become a doctor. Despite all the new technology, students still leave school buried under mountains of debt, experiencing high rates of mental health issues, and frequently underprepared for the real-world pressures of being a doctor.

 It's natural to ask therefore, is the internet truly being utilized to its full potential in the medical space, and just how far can we push this? No doubt many aspects of medical education must remain in person. Students need to see things in three dimensions. They need the steady hand of the professor nearby as they attempt to complete their first dissection. They need the resources and infrastructure that can only be located on a physical campus, including access to cadavers, labs, a library, and the support of their peers.

But a great deal of the process of learning how to be a doctor is rote memorization of facts and processes. This sheer absorption of data can just as easily be done online as it could be in a stuffy lecture hall. At home, students can study in comfort, at less cost, in their own time. This is particularly important for part-time students who need to work to support themselves or who have families to care for.

Add to this the recent breakthroughs in virtual reality, which allow many of the hands-on medical experiences to be conducted without the need for expensive (and corrosive) physical materials. Medical students at the University of California San Francisco are already using "virtual cadavers" to practice anatomy and dissections, rather than relying on recently deceased corpses.

So how can we combine the best of both worlds, giving students the hands-on aspect and the support and resources that come with a physical environment, as well as the flexibility and cost efficiency that come with an online program?

It is not our intention to lay out a full curriculum in this document, but when we phrase the challenge as above, the problem no longer appears insurmountable. The teaching profession may provide some parallel, where online education is mixed with scheduled "hands-on" experiences in the classroom.

Our venerable but aging medical education institutions have only partially embraced the importance of the internet and the power of technology to streamline the education process. If they focused exclusively on the welfare of students and the American healthcare system—in the context of the doctor shortage—they would accept the need to innovate and adapt.

It is possible that the change needed will not come from established institutions that make huge profits, are inundated with applicants, and are comfortable as they are. If a purpose-built, online medical university were sufficiently funded, organized, regulated and established—with the problems outlined above sufficiently addressed—only then may market forces and the laws of competition motivate existing institutions to change.

Lessons from Abroad—How Other Nations Successfully Train and Retain Doctors

The primary, unchangeable cause of the doctor shortage in the United States is a global problem: our aging population. This means that the U.S. is by no means the only country to wrestle with this issue.

Right now, there are already 46 million Americans aged 65 and above. By 2060, this number is expected to double, meaning that almost one quarter of Americans will be over 65. Japan is already there, with its population almost at the point of decline and facing one of the greatest demographic challenges of any developed, industrialized nations.

In China, the demographic challenges are more complicated with factors like the one-child policy putting massive strain on people of working age. With just 189,000 doctors in a country of almost 1.4 billion people, China is in even worse shape than the U.S.

But other countries facing the same challenge have been able to solve this problem, due to more cooperation between the political sector and the education sector, resulting in sufficient numbers of new doctors entering the workforce.

Let's look at an example that may be instructive to the case of the U.S.:

Case Study #1: The Story of Germany

With a population of almost 83 million, Germany is the most populous country in Western Europe. With a highly developed, industrialized economy and a complex national makeup recently shaken up by a massive influx of immigrants, Germany provides an interesting point of comparison with the United States.

As we will see, the fundamental difference between the German and American approaches to healthcare and education is that the German government is willing to take far greater responsibility for the associated expenses, whereas the U.S. still leaves much of the financial burden on the shoulders of individuals and corporations. The German system is also simpler than the American, with students able to begin their medical training immediately after finishing high school, and complete their education within just 6 years, as opposed to up to 14 in the U.S.

Like the U.S. and other developed nations, Germany is facing a major demographic challenge in the form of an aging population. This is a problem that Germany has been battling for almost 5 decades, and the recent additions to the population have helped but not addressed this. As the Federal Statistical Agency puts it, "The decades of imbalances in the age structure of the population remain." Tellingly, death rates have outweighed annual birth rates since 1972, although the one million immigrants who entered the country in 2015 succeeded in bringing the national age of the country down for the first time since the fall of the Berlin Wall in 1989.

From this we see that Germany too must confront the challenge of more people requiring medical care, and fewer people able to provide it. So how does their educational system cope? In Germany the vast majority of medical schools are entirely tax-funded, meaning that unlike the U.S.—where students frequently require $200,000 loans—in Germany, becoming a doctor is free from the student's perspective.

While we are not proposing that the U.S. adopt free medical education too, as strenuously argued above it is clear that America needs to provide more funding for medical education to relieve the burden on students and assist teaching hospitals and other institutions that trainee doctors—and the communities they serve—depend on.

Another critical difference between the German and American medical education systems is the stage at which students begin their training. In the U.S., it is necessary to first acquire a 3-4 year bachelor's degree before entering medical school. In Germany, students are able to begin their medical training right out of high school, and qualify as a doctor within 6 years. It is clear that the German system makes it much quicker and easier to train doctors, removing a a major time-consuming hurdle.

"Germany currently employs an integrated medical curriculum that typically begins right after high school and consists of a 2-year long pre-clinical segment teaching basic sciences and a 4-year clinical segment leading medical students to the practical aspects of medicine. On the other hand, the U.S. education is a two-stage process. After successful completion of a Bachelor's degree in college, an American student goes through a 4-year medical program encompassing 2 years of basic science and 2 years of clinical training."

We can conclude from our brief study of Germany two ways in which the European nation outperforms America:

1. Greater—in fact, almost complete—financial support for students enrolled in medical school.

2. A simpler degree structure meaning in takes less time to become a doctor in Germany than it does in the U.S.

While Germany's system is by no means perfect, we have seen above that if the United States were to take efforts to simplify its medical education process and commit to greater investment in medical education, it would not be walking into unknown territory. It would be following a proven model that has been successful in other wealthy, industrialized Western nations.

Case Study #2: From Third World to First—A Brief Look at Singapore
Singapore is a city-state, a tiny "red dot" on the map in Southeast Asia. An obvious problem of comparison between Singapore and the U.S. is that the population of Singapore is 5.6 million, while the population of the U.S. is 323 million. Clearly, many of the complexities and challenges faced by the American medical system will not find easy parallel in Singapore. Nevertheless, the story of how a small, underdeveloped nation transformed its medical system from virtually nothing into one of the finest in the world during the second half of the 20th century contains some valuable insight.

The first medical school in Singapore was established in 1905. Since Singapore gained independence, first from the British Empire and then from Malaysia in 1965, its economy rapidly took off, with advances in medicine occuring in lockstep with its economic growth. From the earliest stages, the independent government of Singapore took pains to ensure medicine and medical education were a funding priority, resulting in one of the most advanced and successful healthcare and education systems in the world.

Like the U.S. and Germany, Singapore faces a rapidly aging population. As the Singapore Department of Statistics describes the problem, "The proportion of residents aged 65 years and over has increased from 8.5% in 2007 to 13% in 2017. There are now fewer working-age adults to support each resident aged 65 years and over as indicated by the falling resident old-age support ratio from 7.7 in 2007 to 5.1 in 2017."

Looking at the numbers, it is clear that Singapore has the makings of a demographic crisis. But despite the extent of the challenge, they are able to maintain a doctor-to-person ratio of 1:490, ensuring an adequate supply of qualified physicians to meet the ever-growing demand.

As we saw with Germany in the section above, the key to Singapore's success is simple: government investment. "The strong Government support and the establishment have contributed to the success of medical education in Singapore." [Samaraskera, Dujeepa & Ooi, Shirley & Ping Yeo, Su & Hooi, Shing. (2015). Medical education in Singapore. Medical teacher. 37. 1-7. 10.3109/0142159X.2015.1009026.]

The government of Singapore continues to invest in new medical technologies, and ensures that the nation's teaching hospitals and medical universities have access to state-of-the-art equipment. Not for Singapore the crumbling teaching hospital on some abandoned highway. While teaching hospitals are essential—yet often derided or neglected—in the U.S., in Singapore their value to both the short- and long-term needs of the community has always been understood. As the website of Singapore General Hospital explains:

"With the Faculty of Medicine being sited next to the main general hospital, it was inevitable that SGH took on a much heavier load as a teaching hospital.

 University departments were set up in the major disciplines such as Medicine, Surgery and Paediatrics. Students were exposed to every available discipline, and in disciplines without University Departments, such as Ophthalmology, Otolaryngology and Radiology, teaching was carried out by the government departments of the hospital."

A historical commitment to hands-on education that benefits the community, and a persistent willingness to invest government resources in education and medical technology as a priority, has allowed Singapore to develop a first-world medical infrastructure from scratch. It's also helped them maintain a high doctor-patient ratio despite their aging population.

Case Study #3: An Instructive Failure—A Look at Britain's NHS

The examples above look at how two developed economies have successfully overcome their own demographic challenges to create successful—albeit imperfect—healthcare and medical education systems.

Another developed economy that faces similar challenges to the U.S. is Great Britain. In 2018, the headlines were abuzz with reports of chaos at the National Health Service (NHS). Winter and the associated spike in illnesses stretched the resources of the NHS to its limits. When summer came, officials hoped that things would return to normal. However, the high continued, and at the time of writing, the NHS is still suffering.

A closer look at this crisis can be instructive for the purposes of readdressing the state of healthcare and medical education in the United States. The two nations share not only a common language, but political trends tend to be echoed across the Atlantic too;we need only to look at the election of Donald Trump following closely on the heels of Brexit to see an example of this.

Britain's NHS guarantees free healthcare to its 65 million citizens. This has both inspired and infuriated American political commentators from across the pond. When winter and the associated health problems hit the UK in 2018, 150,000 patients had to wait over half an hour at the Accident & Emergency (A&E) ward. In summer, 6.2 million more A&E visits are anticipated, more than 750,000 (that's more than 10%) of whom are expected to face wait times of up to four hours!

For people suffering from horrific injuries and acute illnesses, this is clearly an unacceptable situation. Many will limp away from emergency rooms facing permanent health problems that could have been avoided if the medical attention they so desperately sought had been available when they needed it. "People are dying in the hallways!" a senior consultant told CNN in January, when more than 2 million patients needed NHS care.

While many hoped that the NHS crisis would ease up following the winter strain, the problems are deeply entrenched and seem unlikely to abate. While even the U.S.—with its politically charged opposition to state-funded

healthcare—spends 17.2% of GDP on medical services for its citizens, Britain lags far behind other G7 countries. The spending gap looms large, as reported by the Guardian:
"The [British Medical] Association estimates that health funding in England is more than £7bn a year lower than comparable European countries, and the gap could rise to more than £11bn over the next three years."

When Brexit was sold to the British people, grandiose promises were made that money supposedly shipped off to other European countries would be kept at home and spent to patch up the crumbling NHS. Brexiteers appeared to quickly back away from those promises the moment their unexpected victory occurred.

Instead of increasing funding, the NHS is attempting to pull itself together with "far-fetched" alternatives, such as sending adults to children's wards when crowding exceeds limits. Writing for the Independent, NHS consultant Ravi Jayaram outlines a litany of perils facing the NHS, including the simple fact that hospitals lack even the beds on which to deposit ill patients. He explains that the fundamental issue is that supply has outstripped demand. And yet the problem is not to be blamed on Australian flu, tired doctors or nurses. Jayaram places blame squarely on the political establishment:

"It is entirely down to the Department of Health focusing so much on financial targets that the point of what we are trying to do is being lost. The health service is there for the patients who need it. We seem to be in a situation where the patients have become something of an expensive inconvenience who drain state resources."

Of course, the dire situation in Britain has been seized upon by American lawmakers, eager to point to the disaster as an argument against socialized healthcare. Even Donald Trump chimed in, Tweeting on February 5, 2018: "The Democrats are pushing for Universal HealthCare while thousands of people are marching in the UK because their [Universal] system is going broke and not working. Dems want to greatly raise taxes for really bad and non-personal medical care. No thanks!"

Beyond funding issues, one of the causes of the NHS crisis is the system itself. With the world facing a major doctor shortage, primary care is lacking across Britain—a problem shared by many other developed and developing nations with aging populations.

Instead of a simple primary care visit which could nip a potentially minor health issue in the bud, patients either wait until the problem becomes an emergency, or attend the emergency room anyway, putting their own health at risk and placing further strain on an already overburdened system.

The NHS was founded 70 years ago with a grand principle in mind. Regardless of your age, your wealth, your position in society, you can seek free medical care when you need it the most. But things have changed since 1948. Today,

 18% of Britain's population is aged 65 and older. This means a disproportionate number of people are seeking healthcare compared to those who remain in the workforce and are able to provide it.

We see therefore that the NHS is facing a triple assault: a lack of funds, an aging population, and organization errors have stretched a once venerable institution to the point of collapse. It's not only the patients who are suffering. General practitioners are "on their knees," says Ghislaine Stephenson, a senior pediatric nurse at Whipps Cross University Hospital in East London. Emergency room doctors are going to work in battle-ground conditions, working horrifically long shifts, and coming home exhausted—sometimes in need of medical care themselves!

The Medical World Needs to Adapt to the 21st Century

As with America, so with Britain. If more doctors were able to join the workforce, then a major underlying cause of the catastrophe would be removed. Demand for medical care will continue to increase, so we must act to increase the supply by training more doctors and keeping them healthy, energetic and motivated.

Return to America: Interview with an American Doctor

As you think about the case studies above from Germany, Singapore and Britain, we turn back to America. To emphasize the arguments detailed above and get an insider's perspective on the state of American healthcare, I contacted Cheryl Thieu, Medical Director at the Valley Homeless Healthcare Program in Santa Clara County, California, to get her perspective on the themes in this document.

Here is the conversation below. It is interesting to note that while there are many points of agreement and concurrence with the arguments above, there are points of difference. This serves to highlight the complexity of the issue that we are dealing with, and emphasize the fact that there is no one silver-bullet solution.

Major points of concurrency are on the issues of education and student debt. We have argued above that the need for a bachelor's degree prior to medical school unnecessarily drags out the training process, delaying the arrival of new doctors at a time when the United States desperately needs them. We have also argued about the staggeringly high rates of student loans, and their detrimental effects on the lives of medical students, even long after they become doctors.

Dr. Thieu differs on the issues of an online medical university, which is a bold proposition that the authors expect to generate resistance from the established medical community. We hope that from the arguments presented above, readers will understand why we believe that, though difficult, such a proposition is not as far-fetched as it may at first glance appear.

Interview with Dr. Cheryl Thieu

> Does the United States do enough to financially assist medical students and young doctors?

I think that the U.S. needs to do more to financially support their physicians-in-training. The average medical student debt at the time of graduation is staggering, well over $100K, and now nearing $200K. It is no wonder that we have a shortage of primary care physicians as a student's looming debt surely influences their choice of medical specialty.

> Is the process of becoming a doctor in the United States efficient? What could be changed?

While the value of a liberal arts education at a four-year university is unparalleled, it may not be the best educational route for every future physician. Some physicians-in-training may prefer a shortened training duration, such as some 6-7 year medical programs offered by some universities. Increasing the number of such programs would offer future physicians more options for their training paths that are sensitive to the trainee's personal and career goals.

The World Health Organization estimates that the world is short 7.2 million healthcare workers already, with the primary-care-physician shortage in America set to be as high as 40,000 by 2025. Is this an issue you frequently discuss with your peers? What can be done about it? Are you optimistic that a solution can be found?

This is hot topic of discussion among U.S. physicians. In our current healthcare system, primary care physicians are not provided enough support on a day-to-day basis to meet all the demands expected of them. Our medical system needs to support them in the tasks that prevent them from working at the top of their skill set, such as providing more support in completing paperwork and providing routine healthcare maintenance. Also, there is a stark salary discrepancy / reimbursement difference among primary care physicians and specialists. This needs to be rectified to help meet the workforce demands.

Currently there are no online medical universities. Do you think medicine can be learned online? What are your thoughts about an online medical university?

Medicine has always been a profession that is both an art and a science. Online learning can only provide the science aspect of learning, not the art. It is not a sufficient vehicle to provide a well-trained physician.

Introducing QUPI—Software that Improves Medical Education

We've looked now broadly at the medical education crisis facing America, and examined possible solutions on the government, corporate and education levels. We've seen how other countries are battling with the problem of an aging population and funding their education systems to keep pace. Now we turn away from the context, and zoom in on one specific educational innovation: QUPI.

It's clear that medical education in the United States is in dire need of change. QUPI is a startup company—run by entrepreneurs from the United States, the United Kingdom and Poland—with ambitious plans for reinventing medical education in the 21st century.

In a world of autonomous cars, supersonic jets, high-speed internet, and countless mobile and wireless devices, why are we still teaching medicine the same way we taught it hundreds of years ago? While many startups aim to change the way we study medicine through virtual dissection labs and other ingenious ways, Qupi looks toward a balancing act of learning medicine through the most powerful tool we have, the internet, combined with hands on physical labs at easily accessible physical locations.

Sometimes it takes small innovation to solve big problems. Like the first stone that triggers an avalanche, a small idea can gather pace, inspire others, and eventually result in major disruption. In this vein, QUPI has grown from a simple desktop platform to help medical students study, to an ambitious, millennial-driven organization with plans on radically changing the landscape of medical education in the U.S. and the world.

As the sponsor and distributor of this document, QUPI wants to lay out their vision for transforming medical education in the United States. In that spirit, they have outlined their business plan and vision below:

QUPI Level One: A Question Bank to Help Students Practice Their Medical Knowledge

At its most basic level, QUPI makes it easier for medical students to become doctors.

QUPI began as a medical question bank: a curated list of 10,000 practice questions covering all 12 medical disciplines (Anatomy, Microbiology, Biochemistry, Neurology, Behavioral Science, Pathology, Histology, Physiology, Pharmacology, Pathophysiology, Immunology and Virology). The questions are designed and selected with license exams in mind, designed to equip students with the confidence, thinking skills and knowledge they require to pass tests like the USMLE, NBDE, NBME, MRCP and the MCCQE (for American, British and Canadian students, respectively).

Designed as a desktop platform that students can access online from any computer, QUPI solves a common problem facing medical students around the world: students can acquire knowledge in the classroom, but when it comes to proving this knowledge in a multiple-choice question environment, they fall short. The QUPI app helps bridge this gap and solve this problem by making it easy, fun and convenient to practice medical knowledge in a format that is specifically relevant to university and licensing exams.

QUPI is currently developing a mobile app that will replicate the function of its desktop platform. This means that students will be able to log in on their phones, and enjoy easy and perhaps even "addictive" exam practice wherever they are, be it while waiting in line at a coffee shop, sitting on the subway ride home, or simply relaxing in the living room.

QUPI Level Two: An Integrated Medical Education Platform

At the second level, QUPI aims to replicate the experience of medical school with an integrated online platform available to students around the world. QUPI was created to solve a simple problem faced by many medical students. As happens when you pull a loose thread on an old piece of clothing, once you apply yourself to one problem, you soon learn that it is connected to many others. As described above, there are no online medical universities in the United States. Attending medical school is exceedingly costly, landing students with 6 figures of debt and a wealth of psychological and social issues caused by the huge strain of medical school and the massive amount of associated pressure.

At present, QUPI is in the process of expanding its online presence to create an integrated medical education platform. This will supplement medical students' experiences in established universities; it is not meant to replace them. At least not yet. The online platform will include articles and video lectures by medical experts and enthusiasts, including lectures delivered by me in the style of my popular Future Doc House YouTube channel, (www.youtube.com/user/FutureDocHouse).

QUPI Level Three: The QUPI Legacy Foundation

At the third level, the aims and ambitions of QUPI merge with the earlier content of this document. By mobilizing its advisers and supporters across the United States and by participating in the democratic process, QUPI aims to help reinvent medical education for the 21st century.

This long-term version will require the QUPI app and integrated education platform to gain traction in the United States as well as internationally. Once a critical mass of students and certain revenue targets are reached, QUPI will begin investing in political programs within the United States to attempt to effect positive change on the structure of the U.S. medical education system, in line with the detailed recommendations made earlier in this document.

While other corporations and charities have tried and failed, there are two things that make QUPI different:

1: Proof that online medical education is possible. While QUPI will first exist as a supplement for, rather than a replacement of conventional medical education, the ability to access the latest in medical education and watch lectures streamed from around the world at the click of the button is an irresistible benefit to society as a whole.

When medical knowledge is demystified, unpacked and made available at an affordable price online, conventional medical schools will lose their power and impetus to stifle innovation. QUPI believes that innovation will ultimately triumph against vested interests and conservatism. By ever expanding and adding to its online platform, QUPI will prove this.

2: An organization run by millenials that will not be deterred by the forces of inaction. While QUPI employs many experienced professionals as members of its advisory board, its core leadership team is composed of members of the millennial generation. Their CEO, Damian Ratajczak, is 28 years old. While older companies have been willing to accept the status quo, QUPI will not so easily relent.

It is on the shoulders of the millennial generation that the costs of the doctor shortage will fall. Like an inverted pyramid, the weight of aging generations above them is pushing down on a group that is relatively smaller and smaller. This demographic imbalance will not be solved by the generations that caused this problem, did nothing, and allowed entrenched systems and special interests to stifle innovation. It can only be solved by the generation most affected. This is what makes QUPI different.

How QUPI Is Building Happier, More Well-Rounded Doctors

QUPI distinguishes itself by having on its advisory board not just doctors, but also medical students who are still in the process of completing their studies. Their feedback provides invaluable insights for the medical education industry as a whole on how to build happier, more well-rounded doctors—the kind of doctors who patients actually want!

As we have seen above, medical residents are arriving at their residencies (if they are lucky enough to get them) already burnt out. Often forced to study far from home due to necessity and lack of places, they leave behind their social support structure including their friends and family. Their gruelling schedules mean it's impossible to build a social life from scratch, leading to isolation and depression.

According to the American Foundation of Suicide Prevention, as reported by Vox Media, doctors are between 1.4 and 2.27 more likely to commit suicide than the population as an average. Evidence shows that the problem begins in medical school, where as many as 1 in 3 medical students are affected by depression.

For those who have been through medical school, these statistics are hardly surprising. Advocates like Pamela Wible describe medical school as resembling a military boot camp. Competition is intense, leading to a harsh, cutthroat atmosphere that causes many students to experience disillusionment, burnout and mental health issues.

Those who attend medical school tend to be highly intelligent. This has its benefits but also its costs; those who attend medical school have often breezed through previous schooling without being exposed to the pressure or competition with their fellow best and brightest peers that immediately hits once their medical training begins.

Financial issues exacerbate the problems. As we have seen, students are leaving medical school shackled to horrific amounts of debt, which can hamper them throughout much of their adult lives. Financial burdens become psychological burdens, increasing the already enormous amount of pressure each student has to somehow struggle under.

It has been said that medical schools are entirely to blame, that they themselves cause depression. In an environment where depression is so common, one would hope that help were easy to find. Unfortunately, many students fear that reaching out would jeopardize their future careers, which they of course consider to be of paramount importance.

Nathaniel P. Morris, a medical student at the time at Harvard Medical School, wrote an article about his struggles with depression, and his decision to seek help. Reflecting later in another article in the Washington Post, Morris writes:

"Last spring, I wrote publicly about my own struggle with depression during medical school. The days leading up to the article's publication were terrifying. I worried I might lose the residency slot I had matched into or forfeit the trust of future colleagues. Again and again, I checked the medical licensing requirements in California to make sure I wouldn't lose the ability to care for patients. Yet my fears have gone unfounded and, in the days that followed, I received nothing but support from colleagues and mentors. Fortunately, others are speaking up as well."

It is clear that the medical community needs to be more open. We need to encourage conversation about the pressures faced here, and remove the fear of judgment or adverse consequences that many believe would arise from speaking out.

But beyond this, we need to look at medical education itself.

It's Time to Put the Joy Back into Medical Learning

Being a doctor isn't just about knowledge and technical skills. Patients want happy doctors because they want to feel a connection. Doctors need social skills. They need to listen. They need to have empathy and they need to have compassion. They need to see the whole patient, and leave that patient feeling reassured, uplifted and like they are in safe hands.

Students who succumb to pressure and spend all their time locked up in the library are unlikely to become good doctors. They may acquire a lot of knowledge, but they miss this fantastic opportunity to develop the human, social skills which are just as important in the real world.

Of course the knowledge element is essential. But studying is not everything. Good doctors need to develop into complete, well-rounded individuals. And yes, this means having friends. It means going out occasionally on the weekends. It means playing a sport and pursuing a hobby. And it means not feeling guilty every time they dare lift their weary eyes from the textbooks, and decide to do something fun.

Lasse Hodne is a student in his fifth year at Poznan University of Medical Studies in Poznan. He is the local spokesman for the Norwegian Medical Association, and a member of QUPI's student advisory board.

When asked what he had learned from his five years of study that he wished he'd known sooner, Lasse explained that more than anything else, doctors need to care:

"When you become a doctor, you're going to be pulling 18-hour shifts at the emergency room. Imagine you're exhausted, it's 3 AM at the end of long shift, and a patient comes in, yells at you, acts aggressively, causes problems. Can you see through your frustration and exhaustion and still feel empathy?

"Instead of asking yourself if you're smart enough to be a doctor, ask yourself if you care enough. At the end of an 18-hour shift, can you still find that compassion and manage to motivate yourself to keep doing your job? This level of caring matters far more than raw brainpower, and it will keep you going through the tough times."

The brutal, boot-camp nature of medical school does not create caring doctors. The cutthroat competition and disabling amounts of debt do not create caring doctors. Patients are suffering because doctors are suffering. At a time when the U.S. is desperately short of medical professionals and heading towards a doctor shortage crisis, it's time to put the joy back into medical education.

Technology like QUPI can help reduce the stress of medical school by simply making it easier for students to study in a manner that directly prepares them for their exams. Medical students today are digitally native. Technology is natural and intuitive to them, therefore the information they need in order to pass medical school and practice their medical knowledge should be available in this format. As Lasse Hodne puts it, "My classmates probably spend more time watching video lectures than reading textbooks. We are millennials after all—might as well embrace it!"

How You Can Get Involved to Change Medical Education for the Better

In this document we have seen that medical education in the U.S. is in dire straits. An aging population has put unprecedented strain on the nation's healthcare resources. More and more people require care, but the policy of the U.S. government means that too few doctors are able to qualify, enter the workforce, and provide the care that is required.

We have looked broadly at the changes that need to be made across the government, corporate and education sectors in order to get the U.S. back on track. In summary:

At the Government Level

Outdated government funding restrictions are holding back medical training in the U.S. and preventing new doctors from entering the workforce. We support the AAMC's recommendations:

- To reduce federal caps on residency that are preventing new doctors from entering the workforce.
- To better support and fund public service programs like the National Health Service Corps (NHSC) and Public Service Loan Forgiveness (PSLF) that make it easier for institutions to recruit and retain physicians.

At the Corporate Level

We welcome attempts from corporations to use their wealth and resources to address this problem, but do not believe that an effective, satisfactory solution can come exclusively from the corporate sector.

Selflessness for selfish reasons has encouraged corporations like Amazon, Berkshire Hathaway and JPMorgan Chase, as well as HMOs like Kaiser Permanente, to innovate to provide better healthcare for their employees. We have examined the pros and cons of integrated medical providers like Kaiser and discussed how they can provide more efficient services, but that rural communities are still often left behind.

These efforts are laudable, but without government action to fix the underlying problem, they will not be sufficient to resolve the demographic imbalance and bring enough new doctors into the workforce.

At the Educational Level

 Academic medicine needs to adapt to provide more efficient training, greater benefit to the communities, and reduced financial burden on students. The fact that students leave medical school with an average of $200,000+ in student debt is unacceptable. Too many gifted and hardworking students are put off by the financial burden and long period of study. If the system were streamlined and costs reduced, the U.S. would be able to train more doctors. We support greater flexibility in medical education, with more training moving online, to reduce the costs to the student and taxpayer.

We have seen how teaching hospitals are a shining example of the fusion of medicine and education. Their high-tech facilities provide essential, hard-to-find services to their community, while they educate tomorrow's doctors. Yet teaching hospitals are often misunderstood, underfunded or neglected. We support teaching hospitals.

Your Next Step: Write to Your Representative

If you live in the United States, you can make your voice heard and write to your congressman, emphasizing your support for government action to end the doctor shortage.

In your own words, explain the reasons for your concern, and what action you would like to see taken—for example, reducing federal caps on residency, increasing funding for the NHSC, and exploring the possibility of the creation of the country's first online medical university.

You can find the contact details of your representative online at https://www.house.gov/representatives/find-your-representative

Here is a sample letter, which you are free to adapt and use:

Dear [Representative Joe Bloggs],

I am writing to you as a [citizen / medical student / healthcare professional / patient] concerned about our nation's doctor shortage. As you are probably aware, our aging population means that by 2025, we could be lacking as many as 35,600 primary care physicians, according to the Association of American Medical Colleges (AAMC).

As a member of Congress, you can take a few steps to address this problem. I urge you to follow the recommendations of the AAMC and:

- *Vote to lift federal residency caps, so that more medical students can complete their education and become doctors.*

- *Lend your influence to increase funding for resources like the National Health Service Corps and the Public Service Loan Forgive ness Program, to lift the enormous financial pressure currently endured by medical students.*

With your help, we can ensure America has the healthcare system that it deserves.

Yours sincerely,

[Your Name]

Other Ways to Help—Give a Copy of This Book to a Friend

Despite the many helpful sources in the media, government services and academia that we've drawn upon to create this manifesto, the doctor shortage issue has largely been ignored by the mainstream press. It is easier to increase ratings by covering the latest political scandal, and scare the public with footage of a North Korean missile test, than it is to dissect the truly alarming statistics that have been explored above.

The fact is the United States is heading toward a crisis. If no action is taken, the nation risks a shortage of up to 94,700 physicians by 2025. With doctor wait times already as high as 52 days in urban centers, and rural communities chronically underserved, millions of Americans are missing out on the quality healthcare that should be their right.

You are by now well aware of the problem, but you do not have to be a part of it. By writing to your congressional representative, or distributing this book, or just getting on your soapbox and talking to anyone who will listen, you can be part of the solution.

Visit our website

We have established a charitable foundation to contribute to innovations, influence policy, and do what we can to end the doctor shortage. Our website is http://www.foundation.qupi.com - please visit and leave us your email address so we can keep you informed and up to date.

Conclusion: A Look at How Things Could Be

Remember Jane, the ill woman in rural America, and Jeff, the overworked and overwhelmed medical resident from the introduction? Now that we've explored the problems that lie behind the crisis facing American healthcare and analyzed some possible solutions, let's revisit this scenario from a more optimistic perspective. Instead of a realistic portrait of how the situation stands, let's paint an aspirational image of how things could be if the recommendations and ambitions of this document were fulfilled.

The start of the scene is familiar—Jane is at home in "rural America," and begins to experience shortness of breath and tightness in the chest. However, unlike our previous scenario where her only recourse was to drive a long way to the hospital and wait, shoulder to shoulder with accident victims at a crowded emergency room, things are different.

Because of changes in legislation that have lifted federal residency caps and increased funding for student loan forgiveness, Jane has easy access to primary care physicians much closer to her home. Her doctor is a charming young man called Jeff. Jeff trained in a big city in the next state over but was encouraged due to loan incentives to begin his medical career in this rural district.

Ordinarily at this age, Jeff would merely be an intern, but recent changes in medical education dropped the requirement for medical students to first attain a bachelor's degree. Jeff knew the moment he finished high school that he wanted to be a doctor, so he didn't waste a moment, applying for medical school immediately and beginning to pursue his dream.

Thanks to apps like QUPI that helped Jeff to practice his medical knowledge in a fun and easy way, and a shift in attitude that reduced the pressure and allowed Jeff to grow as a person as well as learning the essential skills of a doctor, his patients love him. They feel understood and genuinely cared for, which in and of itself contributes to his high success rate as a junior doctor.

Jeff has seen Jane frequently over the last few months, and was able to provide her with an early diagnosis of a chronic yet manageable respiratory condition. When Jane begins to experience symptoms, she reaches for the medicine that Jeff has prescribed, has a glass of water, and lies down to rest. Within an hour she is back on her feet and feeling great. No need for a risky journey to town. No additional burden on stretched ER resources. Jane is healthy, and everyone benefits.

America has access to incredible resources, and a level of wealth, education and infrastructure that remains unimaginable for great swathes of the world. The healthcare crisis that America faces is a tragedy that can be avoided, by making intelligent changes in:

- Legislation and government—to distribute funds where they are needed and help combat the impending doctor shortage.

- Corporate attitudes—to harness the resources of our wealthiest corporations to create innovative solutions that benefit the wider communities.

- Education—to increase efficiency, reduce costs and create more well-rounded, happier graduates.

- Technology—to apply the potential of the internet as well as emerg ing technologies across the above sectors, particularly in education.

By doing so, the United States can and will overcome the challenges it faces, and create a healthcare system that better serves patients and medical professionals alike. That is the vision that QUPI puts forward.

Get active

If you like this book and want more books for your family, friends, and colleagues to distribute, please email us at: info@qupi.com

Also visit Our Qupi Legacy Foundation site: **www.foundation.qupi.com** for more ways to get involved.

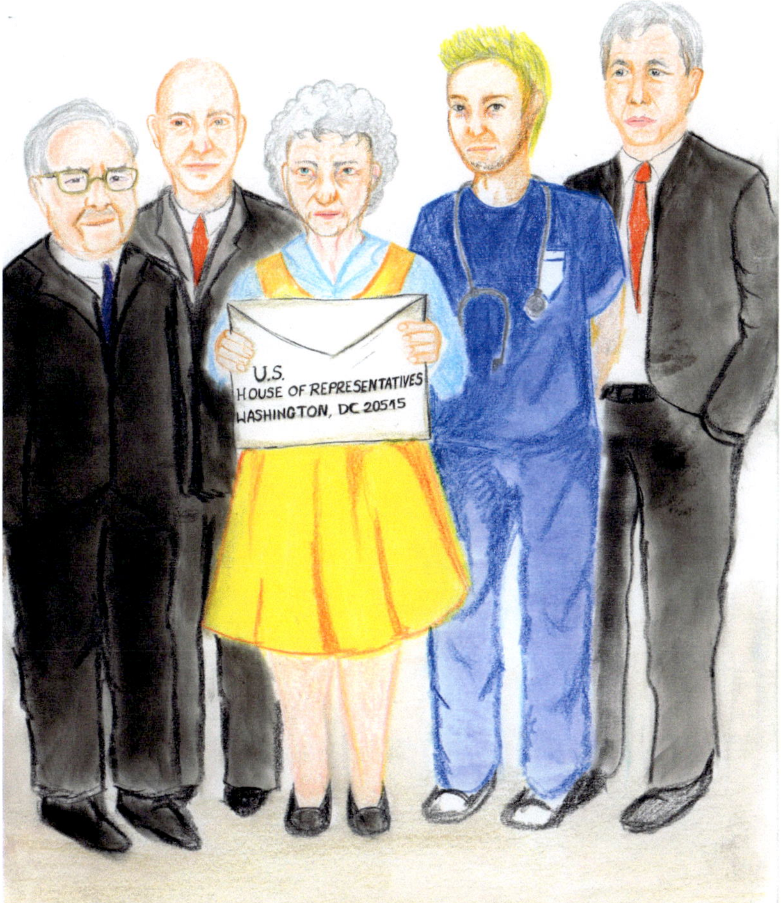
U.S.
HOUSE OF REPRESENTATIVES
WASHINGTON, DC 20515

Made in United States
Cleveland, OH
05 November 2026

47647252R00038